My Thyroid Health

A holistic approach to thyroid conditions

Dr. Frederick Boly

Copyright

TABLE OF CONTENT

Introduction

Welcome to "My Thyroid Health: A Holistic Approach to Thyroid Conditions." by Dr. Frederick Boly. This friendly guide is here to walk you through the world of your thyroid – a small but crucial part of your body that can sometimes throw surprises our way. No need for complicated words; we're keeping it simple, like chatting with a trusted friend.

Chapter 1: Decoding Thyroid Health for Beginners

We'll kick off by understanding what your thyroid does and how it influences your well-being. We'll introduce you to TSH, T3, T4, and decode those common symptoms that might signal something's up. No need for a medical degree – we're breaking it down in everyday language.

Chapter 2: Navigating Thyroid Conditions

Ever felt a bit puzzled about what's happening inside when things feel off? We're diving into the world of thyroid conditions. We'll learn about hypothyroidism, hyperthyroidism, Graves' disease, Hashimoto's, goiter, and thyroiditis. And guess what? We'll understand those numbers on your thyroid report – TSH, T3, and T4. It's like reading a superhero manual for your thyroid.

Chapter 3: Medical Interventions and Advanced Treatments

Now, let's explore superhero treatments. Imagine your thyroid superhero needs a little extra help. We'll talk about thyroidectomy – where a piece or the whole thyroid is removed – and Radioactive Iodine (RAI) – a special treatment to calm an overactive thyroid. We'll check out the good stuff – the advantages – and the not-so-good stuff – the possible side effects. Plus, we'll chat about other superhero treatments for thyroid adventures.

The first three chapters are like building blocks. We'll understand the basics, get to know our thyroid superhero's enemies, and discover ways to help when things go a bit wonky. So far, so good? Now, get ready for the exciting part!

Chapter 4-9: Holistic Approaches for Each Thyroid Adventure

This is where the magic happens. We're going holistic – a fancy word for looking at the whole picture. Each thyroid adventure gets its own special chapter. Hypothyroidism, hyperthyroidism, Graves' disease, Hashimoto's, goiter, and thyroiditis – you get a chapter! We'll explore simple things like what to eat, how to move, and ways to relax for each superhero situation. Real-life stories will make it feel like you're chatting with pals who've been there, done that.

Ready for the journey? Imagine this book as your sidekick, guiding you through the world of thyroid superheroes. No capes needed, just an open heart and a curious mind. Let's dive into "My Thyroid Health" and make your thyroid superhero story one for the books!

Chapter 1

Decoding Thyroid Health for Beginners

In Chapter 1, we're like detectives exploring the mystery of your thyroid. Imagine your thyroid as a tiny superhero in your neck, working hard to keep you feeling good. We'll learn the basics – what the thyroid does and why it's so important. Meet TSH, T3, and T4 – these are like the thyroid's sidekicks, helping it do its job. Together, they influence how you feel and have a big say in your energy levels. We'll keep it simple, so it's like having a chat with a friend who knows all about your thyroid superhero.

Thorough explanation of thyroid gland functions.

Let's break down the thyroid gland's functions in detail. The thyroid is a small, butterfly-shaped gland located in your neck. Its primary role is to produce hormones – thyroxine (T4) and triiodothyronine (T3). These hormones are like messengers that travel through your bloodstream, affecting nearly every cell and organ in your body.

Now, the thyroid doesn't work alone. It takes instructions from the pituitary gland, a tiny gland in your brain. The pituitary gland releases a hormone called thyroid-stimulating hormone (TSH), which signals the thyroid to produce more or less T4 and T3, depending on what your body needs.

The T4 hormone is like a storage form. It's not very active on its own. However, your body can convert some of it into T3, which is the more active and potent hormone. T3 is the one that really gets things moving in your cells, helping with metabolism, energy production, and regulating your body temperature.

Why is all this important? Well, your body's cells need the right amount of T3 to work properly. If there's too much or too little, it can affect your energy levels, mood, weight, and even your heart rate. The thyroid is like a little conductor in an orchestra, ensuring that everything plays in harmony.

But here's the tricky part – the thyroid's balance can be influenced by various factors. Sometimes it produces too much or too little hormone. Conditions like hypothyroidism and hyperthyroidism can result from these imbalances, causing a range of symptoms.

In summary, the thyroid gland is like a master regulator, overseeing the production of hormones that play a crucial role in how your body functions. It's a delicate balance, and when things go awry, it can impact your overall well-being. Understanding this intricate dance of hormones helps us appreciate the thyroid's significance in maintaining good health.

Understanding reference ranges and common symptoms.

Let's take a stroll into the world of reference ranges and common symptoms to decode the language of your body's well-being.

Reference ranges are like the standard measurements for TSH, T3, and T4 levels in your blood. It's a bit like having a thermostat for your thyroid – it helps you know if things are too high, too low, or just right. These ranges may vary slightly between different labs, but they provide a benchmark for what's considered normal.

Now, onto symptoms – these are like your body's signals, telling you when something might be off with your thyroid. For hypothyroidism (when your thyroid is a bit sluggish), common symptoms include feeling tired, gaining weight, and having a sensitivity to the cold. On the flip side, hyperthyroidism (when your thyroid is on overdrive) may show signs like weight loss, restlessness, and feeling too warm.

Think of your body as a messenger. When it senses a thyroid imbalance, it sends signals through these symptoms to catch your attention. Understanding the reference ranges helps your healthcare team interpret these signals more accurately, ensuring you get the right support for your thyroid health journey.

So, reference ranges act as your guideposts, and common symptoms are like gentle nudges from your body, urging you to pay attention. Let's explore these cues together to navigate the fascinating terrain of thyroid well-being.

Overview of additional important thyroid numbers.

Let's expand our exploration beyond TSH, T3, and T4 and introduce some additional important thyroid numbers for a more comprehensive understanding:

1. Free T3 (Triiodothyronine): This is the active form of thyroid hormone, ready to dive into action within your cells. Monitoring free T3 levels provides insights into your body's immediate thyroid activity.

2. Free T4 (Thyroxine): Often called the storage hormone, free T4 is the precursor to T3. Measuring free T4 levels helps assess the thyroid's ability to produce hormones and indicates its potential to convert into the active form.

3. Reverse T3 (rT3): This is like the mirror image of T3 but doesn't have the same superpowers. Elevated levels of reverse T3 may signal that your body is converting too much T4 into this less active form, potentially impacting thyroid function.

4. Thyroglobulin Antibodies (TgAb) and Thyroid Peroxidase Antibodies (TPOAb): These are markers for autoimmune thyroid conditions, such as Hashimoto's disease and Graves' disease. Elevated levels of these antibodies suggest that your immune system may be mistakenly attacking your thyroid.

5. Calcitonin: While not directly related to TSH, T3, or T4, calcitonin levels are crucial for assessing thyroid health, particularly in the context of thyroid cancer. Elevated calcitonin levels may indicate the presence of medullary thyroid cancer.

Chapter 2

Navigating Thyroid Conditions

Welcome to Chapter 2 – "Navigating Thyroid Conditions." This chapter acts as your compass through the varied landscapes of thyroid health. Think of it as a friendly guide helping you understand the different journeys your thyroid might take.

From calm seas like hypothyroidism, where your thyroid takes it easy, to lively currents like hyperthyroidism, making things speed up a bit. We'll explore islands like Graves' disease and Hashimoto's, each with its own unique features. There's also the mountainous challenge of goiter and the ebb and flow of thyroiditis.

In this chapter, we'll navigate through each condition, decoding their signs and making your thyroid adventure a bit less mysterious.

Detailed exploration of common thyroid conditions

1. Hypothyroidism:

- Overview: This is like a gentle slowdown in thyroid activity.
- Causes: Often linked to an underactive thyroid gland or autoimmune disorders like Hashimoto's.
- Symptoms: Fatigue, weight gain, sensitivity to cold, and sluggishness.

2. Hyperthyroidism:

- Overview: Here, the thyroid goes into overdrive.
- Causes: Often associated with an overactive thyroid gland or Graves' disease.
- Symptoms: Restlessness, weight loss, increased heart rate, and feeling too warm.

3. Graves' Disease:

- Overview: An autoimmune condition causing hyperthyroidism.
- Causes: Immune system mistakenly attacks the thyroid, leading to excess hormone production.
- Symptoms: Hyperthyroid symptoms along with possible eye issues like bulging or irritation.

4. Hashimoto's Thyroiditis:

- Overview: An autoimmune condition causing hypothyroidism.

- Causes: Immune system attacks and damages the thyroid, leading to reduced hormone production.
- Symptoms: Hypothyroid symptoms like fatigue, weight gain, and sensitivity to cold.

5. Goiter:
- Overview: Enlargement of the thyroid gland.
- Causes: Can result from iodine deficiency, thyroid nodules, or inflammation.
- Symptoms: Swelling in the neck, difficulty swallowing or breathing.

6. Thyroiditis:
- Overview: Inflammation of the thyroid.
- Causes: Viral or bacterial infections, autoimmune conditions, or medications.
- Symptoms: Fluctuating thyroid function, neck pain, and swelling.

Understanding these conditions involves recognizing their unique characteristics, causes, and symptoms. It's like navigating through different chapters in the thyroid storybook, each presenting its own challenges and solutions.

Interpretation of TSH, T3, T4 levels

1. TSH (Thyroid Stimulating Hormone):
   - Normal Range: 0.4 - 4.0 mIU/L
   - High (Hypothyroidism): > 4.0 mIU/L
   - Low (Hyperthyroidism): < 0.4 mIU/L

2. T3 (Triiodothyronine):
   - Total T3 Normal Range: 80 - 200 ng/dL
   - Free T3 Normal Range: 2.3 - 4.2 pg/mL
   - High (Hyperthyroidism): Levels above the normal range
   - Low (Hypothyroidism): Levels below the normal range

3. T4 (Thyroxine):
   - Total T4 Normal Range: 4.5 - 12.5 µg/dL
   - Free T4 Normal Range: 0.8 - 1.8 ng/dL
   - High (Hyperthyroidism): Levels above the normal range
   - Low (Hypothyroidism): Levels below the normal range

These ranges can vary slightly between laboratories, so it's essential to interpret results in the context of the specific reference ranges provided by the lab that conducted the tests. Always consult with a healthcare professional for a thorough analysis of your results

Comprehensive thyroid panels and autoimmune disorders

A comprehensive thyroid panel typically includes the following tests:

1. TSH (Thyroid Stimulating Hormone): Evaluates overall thyroid function.
2. Free T4 (Thyroxine): Measures the amount of unbound T4 in the blood.
3. Free T3 (Triiodothyronine): Assesses the active thyroid hormone levels.
4. **Total T4 and Total T3**: Measure total levels of these hormones, including both bound and unbound forms.
5. Thyroid Peroxidase Antibodies (TPOAb): Detects antibodies attacking the thyroid, indicating autoimmune thyroid disorders like Hashimoto's thyroiditis.
6. Thyroglobulin Antibodies (TgAb): Tests for antibodies targeting thyroglobulin, another marker for autoimmune thyroid conditions.

7. **Reverse T3 (rT3):** Assesses an inactive form of T3.

If you suspect an autoimmune thyroid disorder, testing for TPOAb and TgAb is crucial. Elevated levels of these antibodies can indicate autoimmune thyroiditis. Consult with a healthcare professional for proper evaluation and interpretation based on your specific health situation.

Additional relevant thyroid markers

In addition to the commonly included markers in a comprehensive thyroid panel, there are other relevant thyroid tests that can provide further insights:

1. **Thyroid-Stimulating Immunoglobulin (TSI):** Detects antibodies that stimulate the thyroid, often elevated in Graves' disease, an autoimmune disorder causing hyperthyroidism.

2. **Thyroid Binding Globulin (TBG):** Evaluates levels of a protein that transports thyroid hormones in the blood, impacting hormone availability.

3. Calcitonin: Measures the hormone produced by the thyroid C-cells, aiding in the diagnosis and monitoring of certain thyroid conditions, such as medullary thyroid cancer.

4. Thyrotropin Receptor Antibodies (TRAb): Similar to TSI, this test can be used to diagnose autoimmune thyroid disorders, particularly Graves' disease.

These additional markers are usually ordered based on specific clinical indications and may not be a routine part of every thyroid panel.

Chapter 3

Medical Interventions and Advanced Treatments

Overview of thyroidectomy, RAI treatments, and other interventions.

Thyroidectomy Overview:
A thyroidectomy is a surgical procedure where the thyroid gland is removed. This can be due to conditions like thyroid cancer, goiter, or hyperthyroidism. Before the surgery, your doctor will likely conduct thyroid function tests, imaging studies, and discuss the risks and benefits with you.

Preparation Tips for Thyroidectomy:
1. Medical Evaluation: Undergo a thorough medical evaluation to ensure you're fit for surgery.
2. Communication: Discuss your medical history, allergies, and medications with your healthcare team.
3. Thyroid Hormone Replacement: Understand the need for thyroid hormone replacement therapy post-surgery and how it will be managed.

21

4. Support System: Arrange for assistance during your recovery, as activities may be restricted initially.

5. Dietary Guidelines: Follow any specific dietary guidelines provided by your doctor, especially if iodine-rich foods need to be restricted.

Radioactive Iodine (RAI) Treatment Overview:
RAI treatment involves ingesting a radioactive form of iodine, targeting and eliminating thyroid cells. It is commonly used for conditions like thyroid cancer.

Preparation Tips for RAI Treatment:

1. Iodine Restriction: Follow instructions to limit iodine-rich foods in the days leading up to treatment.

2. Radiation Safety: Take precautions to minimize radiation exposure to others, especially pregnant women and children.

3. Hydration: Stay well-hydrated to help eliminate radioactive iodine from your body.

Other Interventions Overview:
Besides surgery and RAI, other interventions may include medications like antithyroid drugs or beta-blockers to manage symptoms associated with thyroid disorders.

General Preparation Tips:
1. Follow Instructions: Adhere strictly to any pre-procedure guidelines provided by your healthcare team.
2. Open Communication: Maintain open communication with your doctors and express any concerns.
3. Post-Procedure Care: Understand and prepare for post-surgery or post-treatment care, including possible lifestyle adjustments.
4. Emotional Support: Seek emotional support from friends, family, or support groups if needed.

Advantages , disadvantages, and recovery strategies for thyroidectomy and RAI.

Thyroidectomy:

Advantages:
1. Disease Treatment: Effectively treats thyroid cancer, goiter, and severe hyperthyroidism.
2. Diagnostic Accuracy: Allows for accurate examination of thyroid tissue for cancer or other abnormalities.

Disadvantages:
1. Surgical Risks: Inherent surgical risks such as bleeding, infection, or damage to nearby structures.
2. Hormone Replacement: Lifelong need for thyroid hormone replacement therapy, as the thyroid is removed.

Recovery Strategies:

1. Pain Management:
   - Follow prescribed pain medications.
   - Utilize ice packs or prescribed pain-relief methods to manage discomfort.

2. Thyroid Hormone Replacement Therapy:
   - Adhere to the prescribed thyroid hormone replacement medication to maintain hormonal balance.
   - Regularly monitor thyroid hormone levels through blood tests.

3. Wound Care:
   - Keep the incision area clean and dry.
   - Follow specific wound care instructions provided by your surgeon.

4. Activity Gradual Increase:
  - Gradually resume normal activities to prevent strain.
  - Avoid strenuous exercises initially and consult with your healthcare provider before starting a new exercise regimen.

5. Dietary Considerations:
  - Follow any dietary guidelines provided by your healthcare team.
  - Ensure an adequate intake of nutrients, especially calcium and vitamin D.

6. Emotional Support:
  - Seek emotional support from friends, family, or support groups.
  - Address any concerns or emotional challenges with your healthcare team.

7. Follow-up Appointments:
  - Attend all scheduled follow-up appointments with your surgeon or endocrinologist.
  - Discuss any concerns or questions about your recovery during these visits.

8. Voice Care:

- Be mindful of your voice, as the surgery may affect vocal cords temporarily.
- Avoid excessive talking or whispering during the initial recovery period.

9. Scar Management:
- Follow recommendations for scar management provided by your surgeon.
- Use sunscreen on the scar once it has healed to prevent pigmentation changes.

10. Monitor for Complications:
- Be vigilant for signs of infection, such as increased redness, swelling, or discharge from the incision site.
- Report any unusual symptoms or concerns promptly to your healthcare provider.

Radioactive Iodine (RAI) Treatment:

Advantages:
1. Targeted Treatment: Targets and destroys abnormal thyroid cells without major surgery.
2. Outpatient Procedure: Typically performed as an outpatient procedure.

Disadvantages:

1. Radiation Precautions: Requires precautions to prevent radiation exposure to others.
2. Temporary Worsening of Symptoms: May experience a temporary exacerbation of symptoms before improvement.

Recovery Strategies:
1. Radiation Safety: Follow guidelines to minimize radiation exposure to others.
2. Hydration: Stay well-hydrated to help eliminate radioactive iodine.
3. Symptom Management: Manage temporary worsening of symptoms with medications as prescribed.
4. Follow-up Monitoring: Regularly monitor thyroid function and attend follow-up appointments.

It's crucial to note that individual experiences may vary, and recovery depends on factors like overall health and the specific condition being treated. Discussion of other medical treatments for thyroid-related issues.

Discussion of other medical treatments for thyroid-related issues.

Antithyroid Medications:

Advantages:
1. Non-Invasive: Provides a non-surgical option for managing hyperthyroidism.
2. Hormone Control: Helps regulate excessive thyroid hormone production.

Disadvantages:
1. Relapse Risk: Some may experience a recurrence of hyperthyroidism after discontinuation.
2. Side Effects: Possible side effects, including skin rash or liver issues.

Beta-Blockers:

Advantages:
1. Symptom Relief: Effectively manages symptoms like rapid heart rate and tremors.
2. Adjunct Therapy: Used alongside other treatments for comprehensive symptom control

Disadvantages:
1. Temporary Relief: Provides symptomatic relief but doesn't address the underlying cause.
2. Side Effects: Potential side effects like fatigue or cold extremities.

Levothyroxine (Thyroid Hormone Replacement):

Advantages:
1. Stable Hormone Levels: Ensures stable thyroid hormone levels in cases of hypothyroidism.
2. Oral Administration: Convenient oral administration.

Disadvantages:
1. Lifelong Treatment: Typically requires lifelong use for those with thyroidectomy or hypothyroidism.
2. Dose Adjustments: May need periodic adjustments based on thyroid function tests.

External Beam Radiotherapy:

Advantages:
1. Tumor Control: Used for managing thyroid cancer by targeting cancerous cells.
2. Localized Treatment: Precise targeting of radiation to the affected area.

Disadvantages:
1. Side Effects: Potential side effects like fatigue, skin irritation, or damage to nearby tissues.
2. Multiple Sessions: Treatment often requires multiple sessions.

Alternative Therapies (e.g., Herbal Supplements):

Advantages:
1. Natural Approach: Appeals to those seeking alternative or complementary treatments.
2. Symptom Relief: Some herbs may offer relief for mild symptoms.

Disadvantages:
1. Limited Scientific Evidence: Limited scientific evidence supporting efficacy.
2. Interactions: Potential interactions with medications or inconsistent potency.

Chapter 4

Holistic Approaches to Hypothyroidism

In this chapter, we're exploring different ways to manage hypothyroidism. Instead of just focusing on medicines, we'll look at how lifestyle, emotions, and overall well-being can impact thyroid health. From changing what you eat to finding ways to relax, we'll check out various holistic methods. The goal is to understand how everything connects and find a more complete approach to taking care of your thyroid and yourself. Let's dive into the different aspects that can help make things better in a simple and understandable way.

Dietary strategies, exercise routines, and stress management.

Dietary Strategies for Hypothyroidism:

Foods to Include:

1. Iodine-rich foods: Seafood, dairy, and seaweed to support thyroid function.
2. Selenium sources: Brazil nuts, eggs, and turkey for antioxidant support.
3. Lean proteins: Chicken, fish, beans, and legumes for muscle maintenance.
4. Whole grains: Brown rice, quinoa, and oats for sustained energy.
5. Fruits and vegetables: Rich in vitamins and minerals crucial for overall health.

Foods to Avoid:
1. Soy-based products: May interfere with thyroid hormone absorption.
2. Cruciferous vegetables: Limit intake, especially raw, as they may affect thyroid function.
3. Processed foods: High in sodium and potentially harmful additives.

Recipes:

1. Quinoa Salad:
Ingredients:
- 1 cup quinoa
- 1 cup cherry tomatoes, halved
- 1 cucumber, diced
- 1/2 cup feta cheese, crumbled

- 2 tablespoons olive oil
- 1 lemon, juiced
- Salt and pepper to taste

Instructions:

1. Cook Quinoa: Rinse quinoa under cold water. In a saucepan, combine 1 cup of quinoa with 2 cups of water. Bring to a boil, then reduce heat, cover, and simmer for 15-20 minutes, or until quinoa is cooked and water is absorbed. Fluff with a fork and let it cool.

2. Prepare Vegetables: While quinoa is cooking, chop the cherry tomatoes, dice the cucumber, and crumble the feta cheese.

3. Mix Ingredients: In a large bowl, combine the cooked quinoa, cherry tomatoes, diced cucumber, and crumbled feta cheese.

4. Dress the Salad: In a small bowl, whisk together olive oil, lemon juice, salt, and pepper. Pour the dressing over the quinoa mixture and toss until well combined.

5. Serve: Garnish with additional feta if desired. Serve chilled or at room temperature.

2. Baked Salmon

Ingredients:
- 4 salmon fillets
- 3 cloves garlic, minced
- 1 lemon, juiced
- 2 tablespoons olive oil
- Fresh herbs (e.g., dill, parsley)
- Salt and pepper to taste

Instructions:
1. Preheat Oven: Preheat the oven to 375°F (190°C).

2. Marinate Salmon: In a small bowl, mix minced garlic, lemon juice, olive oil, fresh herbs, salt, and pepper to create the marinade.

3. Coat Salmon: Place salmon fillets in a baking dish and coat them with the marinade, ensuring an even distribution.

4. Bake: Bake in the preheated oven for 15-20 minutes or until the salmon is cooked through and easily flakes with a fork.

5. Serve: Garnish with additional herbs and lemon slices if desired. Serve the baked salmon with your favorite side dishes.

Exercise Routines for Hypothyroidism:

Recommended Exercises:
1. Aerobic exercises: Walking, swimming, or cycling for cardiovascular health.
2. Strength training: Light weights or resistance exercises to maintain muscle mass.
3. Yoga: Promotes flexibility, reduces stress, and supports overall well-being.

Exercises to Avoid:
1. High-impact activities: Intense running or jumping, which may strain joints.
2. Overly strenuous weightlifting: Heavy lifting without proper supervision.
3. Excessive cardio: Long periods of high-intensity cardio, potentially stressing the body.

Stress Management Strategies:

1. Mindfulness Meditation:

- Practice deep-breathing exercises or guided meditation to reduce stress.

2. Regular Breaks:
   - Take short breaks throughout the day to relax and clear your mind.

3. Exercise as Stress Relief:
   - Engage in physical activities as they can help alleviate stress.

4. Balanced Workload:
   - Prioritize tasks and break them into manageable portions to avoid overwhelming stress.

5. Social Support:
   - Connect with friends and family for emotional support.

Importance of sufficient sleep

1. Energy Regulation:
   - Supports the regulation of excess energy associated with hyperthyroidism.
   - Helps manage heightened metabolism and prevent energy depletion.

2. Hormonal Harmony:
- Facilitates the balance of thyroid hormones.
- Adequate sleep may contribute to a more stable hormonal environment.

3. Muscle Repair and Comfort:
- Assists in muscle repair, particularly important as hyperthyroidism can lead to muscle weakness.
- Enhances comfort and reduces physical stress on the body.

4. Cognitive Calmness:
- Supports mental clarity and calmness, counteracting hyperactivity.
- Helps manage anxious thoughts and mental restlessness associated with hyperthyroidism.

5. Immune Support:
- Boosts the immune system, which may be compromised in hyperthyroid conditions.
- Supports the body's ability to fight infections and maintain overall health.

6. Emotional Equilibrium:
- Contributes to emotional balance and stress reduction.

- Important for individuals with hyperthyroidism who may experience heightened emotions.

7. Heart Health:
- Supports cardiovascular health by regulating heart rate.
- Reduces the strain on the heart, which can be increased in hyperthyroidism.

8. Weight Management:
- Facilitates weight management by influencing appetite-regulating hormones.
- Helps prevent unintentional weight loss often associated with hyperthyroidism.

9. Thyroid Function Support:
- Plays a role in supporting the overall function of the thyroid gland.
- Contributes to maintaining a more stable thyroid environment.

10. Overall Well-being:
- Enhances overall well-being and quality of life for individuals with hyperthyroidism.
- Promotes a sense of balance and resilience.

Ensuring sufficient sleep is a valuable component in managing the symptoms and promoting well-being for individuals dealing with hyperthyroidism.

Natural herbs

1. Bugleweed (Lycopus virginicus):
- Description: Bugleweed is an herbaceous plant traditionally used to manage hyperthyroid symptoms.
- How to Use: Prepare bugleweed tea by steeping 1 teaspoon of dried leaves in hot water for 5-10 minutes. Consume up to three times a day.

2. Lemon Balm (Melissa officinalis):
- Description: Lemon balm, known for its calming properties, is believed to help with hyperthyroidism symptoms.
- How to Use: Make lemon balm tea by steeping 1-2 teaspoons of dried leaves in hot water. Drink 2-3 cups per day.

3. Motherwort (Leonurus cardiaca):
- Description: Motherwort has a long history in traditional medicine for thyroid support and stress reduction.

- How to Use: Prepare motherwort tea by steeping 1-2 teaspoons of dried leaves in hot water. Drink up to three times daily.

4. Ashwagandha (Withania somnifera)
   - Description: Ashwagandha, an adaptogenic herb, may help balance thyroid function and reduce stress.
   - How to Use: Consume ashwagandha supplements as per the recommended dosage on the product packaging.

5. Siberian Ginseng (Eleutherococcus senticosus):
   - Description: Known as an adaptogen, Siberian ginseng may support the body's response to stress, often associated with hyperthyroidism.
   - How to Use: Take Siberian ginseng supplements following the recommended dosage.

6. Evening Primrose Oil (Oenothera biennis):
   - Description: Evening primrose oil contains gamma-linolenic acid, believed to help regulate thyroid function.
   - How to Use: Consume evening primrose oil supplements according to the product instructions.

7. Guggul (Commiphora wightii):

- Description: Guggul has been used in traditional Ayurvedic medicine for thyroid support.
- How to Use: Take guggul supplements following the recommended dosage.

8. Bladderwrack (Fucus vesiculosus):

- Description: Rich in iodine, bladderwrack is considered for thyroid support.
- How to Use: Typically available in supplement form; follow the recommended dosage.

9. Nettle (Urtica dioica):

- Description: Nettle is rich in minerals and may support overall thyroid health.
- How to Use: Prepare nettle tea by steeping 1-2 teaspoons of dried leaves in hot water. Consume up to three times a day.

While these herbs are often considered for thyroid support, it's crucial to consult with a healthcare professional before incorporating them into your routine, especially if you are already on medication or have pre-existing health conditions. Herbs may interact with medications or have contraindications for certain individuals. Always prioritize safety and informed decision-making regarding your health.

Managing Symptoms

Let's delve into practical solutions for managing hypothyroidism symptoms, explaining why each approach can be beneficial in simple terms:

1. Fatigue:

- Quality Sleep: Adequate and consistent sleep is like recharging your body's batteries. It gives your thyroid hormones a chance to do their job, boosting energy levels.

- B-Vitamin-Rich Foods: Foods like meat, eggs, and leafy greens are like fuel for your body. They contain B-vitamins that help turn the food you eat into energy.

- Coenzyme Q10 Supplements: Think of these supplements as helpers that support your body's energy production. They provide an extra boost for those times when fatigue feels overwhelming.

2. Weight Gain:

- Balanced Diet: Imagine your body as a car. A balanced diet with a mix of different foods is like giving the right kind of fuel to your body's engine, helping it burn calories efficiently.

- Regular Exercise: Exercise is like revving up the engine. It makes your body burn more calories, helping you maintain a healthy weight.

-CLA Supplements: These are like additional helpers that may support your body in managing weight. They work alongside your efforts to maintain a healthy balance.

3. Sensitivity to Cold:

- Dress in Layers: Imagine putting on a cozy jacket or wrapping yourself in a warm blanket. Dressing in layers is like creating a shield against the cold, helping your body stay comfortably warm.

- Iron-Rich Foods: Foods like lean meats and leafy greens provide your body with iron, which is like a little heater for your blood. It helps keep you warm from the inside.

- Thermogenic Spices: Spices like cayenne pepper or ginger are like turning up the heat in your body. They have properties that can make you feel warmer.

4. Dry Skin and Hair Loss:

- Stay Hydrated: Drinking enough water is like giving your body a drink of freshness. It keeps your skin hydrated and your hair moisturized.

- Use Moisturizers: Moisturizers act like a protective shield for your skin. They lock in moisture, preventing dryness and itching.

- Omega-3 Fatty Acid Supplements: These supplements are like giving your hair a nourishing treat. They provide essential nutrients that support healthy, strong hair

- Folate Supplements: Folate is involved in cell division and replication and plays an important role in hair growth. Supplementing with folate rich diets like leafy greens and legumes would help hair growth. Folate is also most gotten from Vit B. Complex supplements too

5. Changes in Menstrual Patterns:

- Maintain a Healthy Lifestyle: Picture a balanced scale. Keeping a healthy weight and lifestyle helps balance your body's hormones, supporting regular menstrual cycles.

- Zinc-Rich Foods: Foods like pumpkin seeds are like tiny helpers for your hormones. They provide zinc, which plays a role in keeping your hormonal balance in check.

- Chaste Tree Supplements: These supplements are like assistants for your menstrual cycle. They may help in managing irregularities, but it's important to consult with a professional before adding them.

Chapter 5

Holistic Approaches to Hyperthyroidism

Welcome to Chapter 5: Holistic Approaches to Hyperthyroidism. In this chapter, we'll explore simple and wholesome ways to bring balance to an overactive thyroid. Think of it as a guide filled with practical tips and natural strategies to help your body find its calm and harmony when dealing with hyperthyroidism. Let's dive into a world of holistic approaches that work together to support your well-being and promote a healthier thyroid.

Dietary recommendations

Foods to Eat for Managing Hyperthyroidism:

1. Lean Proteins: Think of lean meats, poultry, and fish as your thyroid's allies. They provide essential

amino acids for overall health and support muscle function.

2. Whole Grains: Foods like brown rice and whole wheat are like slow-burning energy sources. They help stabilize blood sugar levels and provide a steady release of energy.

3. Fruits and Vegetables: Colorful fruits and veggies are like a nutrient treasure chest. They offer vitamins, minerals, and antioxidants that contribute to overall health and support the immune system.

4. Dairy or Dairy Alternatives: Calcium and vitamin D from sources like milk or fortified plant-based alternatives are like building blocks for strong bones and can help balance the effects of hyperthyroidism on bone health.

5. Nuts and Seeds: These are like tiny powerhouses. They contain healthy fats, vitamins, and minerals that can support thyroid function.

Foods to Limit or Avoid:

1. Iodine-Rich Foods: While iodine is crucial for thyroid health, too much can be like adding fuel to

the fire in hyperthyroidism. Limit foods like seaweed, iodized salt, and certain seafood.

2. Caffeine: Imagine caffeine as a stimulant, like pressing the gas pedal for your body. In hyperthyroidism, it's like giving an already speedy engine an extra boost. Consider limiting caffeine intake.

3. Sugary Foods: These are like a quick burst of energy that doesn't last. They can contribute to blood sugar fluctuations, which may not be ideal for managing hyperthyroidism symptoms.

4. Processed Foods: Think of heavily processed foods as having too many ingredients your body doesn't need. They often contain additives that might not be supportive of overall health.

5. Soy Products: While small amounts are usually fine, large quantities of soy can interfere with thyroid hormone absorption. It's like a little roadblock for your thyroid function.

Foods that are generally good for both hyper and hypothyroidism

1. Lean Proteins: Sources like chicken, fish, and lean meats are generally beneficial for both conditions, providing essential amino acids.

2. Fruits and Vegetables: Colorful fruits and veggies offer a variety of vitamins, minerals, and antioxidants that support overall health and may be beneficial for both hyperthyroidism and hypothyroidism.

3. Nuts and Seeds: These are rich in healthy fats, vitamins, and minerals, contributing to overall thyroid health.

4. Whole Grains: Opting for whole grains like brown rice, oats, and whole wheat provides a steady source of energy and fiber, which can be supportive for both conditions.

Recipes

1. Grilled Chicken and Vegetable Stir-Fry:

Ingredients:
- Chicken breast strips
- Broccoli florets
- Bell peppers (sliced)

49

- Snap peas
- Carrots (julienned)
- Ginger and garlic (minced)
- Soy sauce
- Sesame oil
- Olive oil
- Brown rice (optional, for serving)

Instructions:
1. Stir-fry chicken in olive oil until cooked.
2. Add ginger and garlic, then toss in vegetables.
3. Pour soy sauce and sesame oil over the mixture, cooking until veggies are tender-crisp.
4. Serve over brown rice if desired.

2. Baked Cod with Sweet Potato and Asparagus

Ingredients:
- Cod fillets
- Sweet potatoes (sliced)
- Asparagus spears
- Lemon juice
- Olive oil
- Paprika
- Salt and pepper

Instructions:

1. Preheat the oven and place cod on a baking sheet.
2. Arrange sweet potato slices and asparagus around the cod.
3. Drizzle with olive oil, lemon juice, and sprinkle with paprika, salt, and pepper.
4. Bake until the cod flakes easily and vegetables are tender.

3. Lentil and Spinach Curry:

Ingredients:
- Green or brown lentils
- Spinach leaves
- Onion (chopped)
- Tomatoes (diced)
- Curry powder
- Cumin and coriander powder
- Garlic and ginger (minced)
- Coconut milk
- Olive oil
- Rice (for serving)

Instructions:
1. Cook lentils until tender.
2. Sauté onions, garlic, and ginger in olive oil until golden.

51

3. Add tomatoes, curry powder, cumin, and coriander; cook until tomatoes are soft.
4. Stir in cooked lentils, spinach, and coconut milk. Simmer until spinach wilts.
5. Serve the lentil curry over rice.

Exercises for Hypothyroidism

Calming exercises for managing hyperthyroidism

1. Walking:
   Take a good walk for about 20-30 minutes. Stand up straight, swing your arms, and wear comfy shoes.

2. Swimming:
   Swim in a pool for a bit. Start slow, maybe with freestyle or breaststroke. Don't forget to breathe and rest when needed.

3. Cycling:
   Ride a bike, either stationary or outdoors. Begin at a medium speed for 20-30 minutes. Sit up straight, and adjust the difficulty level as you feel comfy.

4. *Strength Training
   Lift moderate weights 2-3 times a week. Do exercises like squats or bicep curls. Start with a weight that's a bit challenging but lets you control your movements. Increase it slowly.

5. Yoga:
   Try easy yoga poses like Child's Pose or Legs Up the Wall. For Child's Pose, sit back on your heels and stretch your arms forward. For Legs Up the Wall, lie on your back with legs against a wall. Hold these poses for 5-10 minutes, and focus on taking deep breaths.

Exercises to avoid

For those dealing with hyperthyroidism, it's advisable to avoid exercises that may overly strain the body or exacerbate symptoms. Here are some activities to be cautious about:

1. High-Intensity Cardio:
   Skip intense activities like sprinting or high-impact aerobics, as they can increase heart rate significantly.

2. Excessive Weightlifting:

Avoid lifting extremely heavy weights, as this could strain your muscles and might not be suitable for individuals with hyperthyroidism.

3. Hot Yoga or Hot Workouts:
Steer clear of exercises done in very hot environments, as hyperthyroidism can affect how your body regulates temperature.

4. Extended Endurance Exercises:
Long-distance running or prolonged endurance activities may put excessive stress on the body, so it's wise to keep these in moderation.

5. Strenuous Inversions:
While yoga is generally beneficial, be cautious with intense inversions like headstands or shoulder stands, as they may impact thyroid function.

Strategies for managing insomnia

1. Establish a Consistent Sleep Schedule:
- Go to bed and wake up at the same time every day, even on weekends. This helps regulate your body's internal clock.

2. Create a Relaxing Bedtime Routine:
   - Engage in calming activities before bedtime, such as reading, taking a warm bath, or practicing relaxation techniques. This signals to your body that it's time to wind down.

3. Optimize Your Sleep Environment:
   - Keep your bedroom dark, quiet, and cool. Use blackout curtains, earplugs, or a white noise machine if needed. Invest in a comfortable mattress and pillows.

4. Limit Exposure to Screens Before Bed:
   - Reduce exposure to blue light from phones, tablets, and computers at least an hour before bedtime. The light emitted can interfere with the production of the sleep hormone melatonin.

5. Watch Your Diet:
   - Avoid large meals, caffeine, and nicotine close to bedtime. Opt for a light snack if you're hungry before sleep.

6. Get Regular Exercise
   - Engage in regular physical activity, but try to finish exercising at least a few hours before

bedtime. Exercise can promote better sleep, but doing it too close to bedtime may have the opposite effect.

7. Manage Stress:
   - Practice stress-reducing techniques such as deep breathing, meditation, or progressive muscle relaxation. Consider keeping a journal to jot down any worries before bedtime.

8. Limit Naps:
   - If you nap during the day, keep it short (20-30 minutes) and avoid napping late in e day, as it may interfere with nighttime sleep.

9. Restrict Stimulants:
   - Cut back on stimulants like caffeine and nicotine, especially in the afternoon and evening.

10. Consider Cognitive Behavioral Therapy for Insomnia (CBT-I):
   - CBT-I is a structured program that helps address thoughts and behaviors that hinder sleep. It's an effective, evidence-based approach for managing insomnia.

11. Evaluate Medication Use:

- If insomnia persists, consult a healthcare professional. They may explore medications in certain situations, but these are often considered after non-pharmacological interventions.

Natural herbs

1. Hawthorn (Crataegus spp.):
- How it Works: Hawthorn has cardiovascular benefits and may help alleviate symptoms such as palpitations associated with hyperthyroidism.
- How to Use: Often consumed as an herbal tea or in supplement form. Dosages should be discussed with a healthcare professional.

2. Pasque Flower (Pulsatilla vulgaris):
- How it Works: Pasque flower has been traditionally used for its calming effects and may help with anxiety and restlessness associated with hyperthyroidism.
- How to Use: Typically consumed as an herbal tea or in homeopathic preparations. Dosages should be determined with input from a healthcare professional.

3. Ginger (Zingiber officinale):
   - How it Works: Ginger has anti-inflammatory properties and may provide relief for symptoms like joint pain associated with certain hyperthyroid conditions.
   - How to Use: Often consumed in cooking or as a tea. Ginger supplements are also available. Dosages should be discussed with a healthcare professional.

4. Astragalus (Astragalus membranaceus):
   - How it Works: Astragalus is an adaptogenic herb that may help modulate the immune system and support overall health.
   - How to Use: Typically available in supplement form. Dosages should be determined with input from a healthcare professional.

5. Bugbane (Cimicifuga racemosa):
   - How it Works: Bugbane, also known as black cohosh, has anti-inflammatory properties and may help manage symptoms associated with hyperthyroidism.
   - How to Use: Available in supplement form or as an herbal tea. Dosages should be discussed with a healthcare professional.

As with any herbal remedies, it's crucial to approach them with caution and under the guidance of a healthcare professional, especially when managing conditions like hyperthyroidism. These herbs should complement, not replace, conventional medical care, and regular communication with your healthcare provider is essential.

Managing Symptoms

1.Rapid Heartbeat (Palpitations):

Management:

 - Stay Calm: Take a deep breath and try to stay calm. Anxiety can exacerbate palpitations.

- Deep Breathing: Practice deep breathing exercises. Inhale slowly through your nose, hold for a few seconds, and then exhale slowly through your mouth. Focus on your breath to help calm your nervous system.

- Relaxation Techniques: Engage in relaxation techniques such as meditation or guided imagery.

Visualize a calming scene or use imagery that brings a sense of tranquility.

- Change Positions: Try changing your body position. Sometimes, standing up and moving around can influence blood flow and help alleviate palpitations.

- Splash Cold Water: Splash your face with cold water or take a cool shower. The sensation of cold water can have a calming effect on the nervous system.

- Cough or Valsalva Maneuver: If you feel comfortable doing so, try coughing or performing the Valsalva maneuver. These actions can sometimes stimulate the vagus nerve and regulate heart rhythm.

- Avoid Triggers: Identify and avoid known triggers, such as caffeine or stressful situations, as much as possible.

- Seek Support: If palpitations persist or are causing significant distress, seek support from friends, family, or colleagues. Sometimes, talking about your feelings can help alleviate anxiety.

2. Anxiety and Nervousness:
  - Management:
  - Practice stress management techniques, including regular exercise.
  - Consider herbal supplements like lemon balm, under professional guidance.
  - Attend counseling or support groups if needed.

3.Weight Loss:
  - Management:
  - Ensure a nutrient-dense, balanced diet to maintain adequate calorie intake.
  - Work with a dietitian to address specific nutritional needs.
  - Regularly monitor weight changes and report them to your healthcare provider.

4. Fatigue:
  - Management:
    - Prioritize sufficient and quality sleep.
    - Plan rest periods throughout the day.
    - Adjust daily activities to avoid overexertion.

5. Heat Intolerance and Sweating:
  - Management:
    - Wear lightweight, breathable clothing.

- Use fans or cool compresses to stay comfortable.

- Avoid excessive exposure to heat.

6. Tremors and Shaky Hands:
- Management:

- Deep Breathing: Take slow, deep breaths. Inhale deeply through your nose, hold for a few seconds, and exhale slowly through your mouth. Focus on your breath to help calm your nervous system.

- Hold a Stable Object: Hold onto a stable object or surface, such as a table or countertop. This can provide support and help steady your hands.

- Gentle Stretching: Gently stretch your hands and fingers. Open and close your fists, and perform slow, controlled hand movements to help improve coordination.

- Relaxation Techniques: Engage in relaxation techniques, such as progressive muscle relaxation. Start by tensing and then slowly relaxing different muscle groups in your body.

- Temperature Adjustment: Adjust the temperature in your environment. Sometimes, extreme temperatures, whether too hot or too cold, can impact tremors.

- Change Your Focus: Redirect your attention to another task or activity. Engaging in a different activity may shift your focus and reduce anxiety-related tremors.

- Stay Hydrated: Ensure you are well-hydrated. Dehydration can sometimes exacerbate tremors.

- Wait It Out: Sometimes, tremors may be temporary. Take a moment to wait and observe if the symptoms subside on their own.

- Avoid Stimulants: If you've recently consumed stimulants like caffeine, consider avoiding them in the moment, as they can contribute to increased tremors.

- Supportive Posture: Maintain a supportive posture. Sit or stand in a way that feels stable, and avoid positions that may increase shakiness.

7. Increased Bowel Movements:

- Management:**ll

    - Maintain a fiber-rich diet for digestive health.

    - Stay hydrated.

    - Report any significant changes to your healthcare provider.

9. Enlarged Thyroid (Goiter):

- Management:

    - Follow your healthcare professional's prescribed treatment plan.

    - Monitor thyroid function regularly.

10. Eye Changes (Graves' Ophthalmopathy):

- Management:

    - Consult an eye specialist for management strategies.

    - Use lubricating eye drops for dry eyes.

    - Manage stress to help minimize eye-related symptoms.

Chapter 6

Holistic Approaches to Grave's

Chapter 6 is where we break away from hyperthyroidism and hypothyroidism. Buckle up as we dive into the intriguing realm of Grave's disease – a cool twist to our exploration in holistic approaches.

Anti-inflammatory diet

An anti-inflammatory diet for Graves' disease aims to reduce inflammation and support overall well-being. Here are general guidelines on what to include and avoid:

Foods to Include:

1. Fruits and Vegetables:
   - Rich in antioxidants and phytochemicals, fruits and vegetables help combat inflammation. Aim for a

variety of colors to ensure a diverse range of nutrients.

2. Fatty Fish:
  - Cold-water fish like salmon, mackerel, and sardines contain omega-3 fatty acids, known for their anti-inflammatory properties.

3. Whole Grains
  - Opt for whole grains like brown rice, quinoa, and oats, which provide fiber and nutrients without causing rapid spikes in blood sugar.

4. Lean Proteins:
  - Choose lean protein sources such as poultry, fish, legumes, and tofu. These provide essential amino acids without excess saturated fat.

5. Nuts and Seeds:
  - Almonds, walnuts, flaxseeds, and chia seeds are rich in healthy fats and antioxidants.

6. Healthy Fats:
  - Include sources of healthy fats like avocados and olive oil. These fats have anti-inflammatory effects.

7. Probiotic-Rich Foods:
   - Yogurt, kefir, sauerkraut, and other fermented foods can support gut health, influencing the immune system and inflammation.

8. Herbs and Spices:
   - Turmeric, ginger, garlic, and other herbs and spices have anti-inflammatory properties.

9. Green Tea:
   - Green tea contains polyphenols with antioxidant and anti-inflammatory effects.

Foods to Limit or Avoid:

1. Iodine-Rich Foods:
   - Excessive iodine intake can exacerbate hyperthyroidism. Limit iodine-rich foods like seaweed, iodized salt, and certain seafood.

2. Processed Foods:
   - Processed and refined foods often contain additives and trans fats that may contribute to inflammation. Minimize the intake of packaged snacks and fast food.

3. Sugary Foods and Beverages:

- High sugar consumption can lead to inflammation. Reduce intake of sugary snacks, sodas, and desserts.

4. Gluten:
   - Some individuals with autoimmune conditions find benefits in reducing or eliminating gluten-containing foods. Consider trying a gluten-free diet and monitor its impact on symptoms.

5. Dairy:
   - Dairy may trigger inflammation in some people. Experiment with reducing or eliminating dairy products and opting for dairy alternatives if needed.

6. Red and Processed Meat:
   - Limit the intake of red and processed meats, as they can contribute to inflammation. Opt for leaner protein sources.

7. Alcohol:
   - Excessive alcohol consumption can contribute to inflammation. Consume alcohol in moderation or consider abstaining.

Recipes for Grave's patients

Here are some food recipes that incorporate ingredients known for their potential anti-inflammatory and nutrient-rich properties, which may be beneficial for those with Graves' disease.

1. Salmon and Quinoa Bowl:

Ingredients:
- 1 cup cooked quinoa
- Grilled or baked salmon fillets
- Mixed greens (spinach, kale, arugula)
- Cherry tomatoes, halved
- Cucumber, sliced
- Avocado, sliced
- Olive oil and lemon dressing

Instructions:
1. Cook quinoa according to package instructions.
2. Grill or bake salmon fillets until cooked through.
3. Assemble bowls with quinoa as the base, topped with mixed greens, cherry tomatoes, cucumber, avocado, and salmon.
4. Drizzle with olive oil and lemon dressing.

2. Vegetarian Stir-Fry with Tofu:

Ingredients:
- Firm tofu, cubed

- Broccoli florets
- Bell peppers, sliced
- Carrots, julienned
- Snap peas
- Garlic and ginger, minced
- Low-sodium soy sauce
- Sesame oil
- Brown rice or quinoa (optional)

Instructions:
1. Press excess water from tofu and cut into cubes.
2. Stir-fry tofu until golden brown.
3. Add garlic and ginger, then stir in broccoli, bell peppers, carrots, and snap peas.
4. Drizzle with low-sodium soy sauce and sesame oil.
5. Serve over brown rice or quinoa if desired.

3. Turmeric Chickpea Curry:
Ingredients:
- Chickpeas, cooked or canned
- Onion, finely chopped
- Garlic and ginger, minced
- Tomatoes, diced
- Spinach or kale, chopped
- Turmeric, cumin, coriander, and paprika
- Coconut milk

- Basmati rice

Instructions:
1. Sauté onions, garlic, and ginger until softened.
2. Add turmeric, cumin, coriander, and paprika, stirring to combine.
3. Stir in diced tomatoes and cooked chickpeas.
4. Pour in coconut milk and simmer until flavors meld.
5. Add chopped spinach or kale and cook until wilted.
6. Serve over basmati rice.

4. Quinoa and Vegetable Stuffed Bell Peppers:
Ingredients:
- *Bell peppers,* halved
- Cooked quinoa
- Black beans, drained and rinsed
- Corn kernels
- Diced tomatoes
- Red onion, finely chopped
- Cumin, chili powder, and garlic powder
- Shredded cheese (optional)

Instructions:
1. Preheat the oven to 375°F (190°C).

2. In a bowl, mix cooked quinoa, black beans, corn, diced tomatoes, red onion, and season with cumin, chili powder, and garlic powder.

3. Stuff each bell pepper half with the quinoa mixture.

4. If desired, sprinkle shredded cheese on top.

5. Bake for 20-25 minutes until peppers are tender.

5. Lentil and Vegetable Soup:

Ingredients:
- Green or brown lentils, rinsed
- Carrots, diced
- Celery, chopped
- Onion, finely chopped
- Garlic, minced
- Vegetable broth
- Tomatoes, diced
- Spinach or kale, chopped
- Turmeric, thyme, and bay leaves

Instructions:
1. In a large pot, sauté onion and garlic until softened.

2. Add lentils, carrots, celery, tomatoes, vegetable broth, turmeric, thyme, and bay leaves.

3. Bring to a boil, then reduce heat and simmer until lentils are cooked.

4. Stir in chopped spinach or kale before serving.

6. Grilled Chicken and Avocado Salad:
Ingredients:
- Grilled chicken breast, sliced
- Mixed salad greens (arugula, spinach, watercress)
- Avocado, sliced
- Cherry tomatoes, halved
- Cucumber, sliced
- Balsamic vinaigrette dressing

Instructions:
1. Grill chicken breast until fully cooked, then slice.
2. In a large bowl, combine mixed salad greens, avocado slices, cherry tomatoes, and cucumber.
3. Top with sliced grilled chicken.
4. Drizzle with balsamic vinaigrette dressing before serving.

7. Mango and Black Bean Salad:
Ingredients:
- Black beans, drained and rinsed
- Mango, diced
- Red bell pepper, chopped
- Red onion, finely sliced
- Cilantro, chopped
- Lime juice

- Olive oil
- Salt and pepper

Instructions:
1. In a bowl, combine black beans, diced mango, chopped red bell pepper, and sliced red onion.
2. In a separate small bowl, whisk together lime juice, olive oil, salt, and pepper to create the dressing.
3. Pour the dressing over the salad and toss gently.
4. Garnish with chopped cilantro before serving.

8. Turkey and Vegetable Stir-Fry:
Ingredients:
- Ground turkey
- Broccoli florets
- Carrots, sliced
- Snap peas
- Garlic and ginger, minced
- Low-sodium soy sauce
- Sesame oil
- Brown rice or cauliflower rice (for a low-carb option)

Instructions:
1. In a wok or skillet, cook ground turkey until browned.

2. Add garlic and ginger, then stir in broccoli, carrots, and snap peas.

3. Drizzle with low-sodium soy sauce and sesame oil.

4. Cook until vegetables are tender yet still crisp.

5. Serve over brown rice or cauliflower rice.

Feel free to adapt these recipes to your taste preferences and dietary requirements.

Balanced exercise and stress relief

Recommended Exercises:

1. Low-Impact Cardio:
   - Engage in activities like brisk walking, cycling, or swimming for cardiovascular health without placing excessive stress on joints.

2. Yoga:
   - Incorporate yoga for flexibility, balance, and relaxation. Choose gentle or restorative yoga classes.

3. Strength Training:

- Include light to moderate strength training using resistance bands or bodyweight exercises to maintain muscle tone.

4. Mind-Body Practices:
   - Explore mind-body activities such as tai chi or qigong for a combination of movement and relaxation.

Exercises to Avoid:
1. High-Impact Cardio:
   - Steer clear of high-impact activities like running or intense aerobics, as they may put additional strain on the body.

2. Heavy Weightlifting:
   - Avoid heavy weightlifting, especially if it causes excessive strain or fatigue.

3. Overly Intense Workouts:
   - Be cautious with overly intense workouts that may lead to exhaustion and negatively impact the adrenal glands.

Importance of Stress Relief for Graves:

1. Impact on Hyperthyroidism:

- Chronic stress can exacerbate hyperthyroid symptoms. Stress activates the body's fight-or-flight response, potentially worsening the overactive thyroid function.

2. Immune System Support:
   - Stress weakens the immune system, and individuals with Graves' disease have an autoimmune component. Managing stress helps support the immune system.

3. Hormone Balance:
   - Chronic stress can disrupt hormone balance, including thyroid hormones. Stress relief practices contribute to hormonal equilibrium.

4. Quality of Life:
   - Stress management enhances overall well-being, helping individuals with Graves' disease lead a more balanced and fulfilling life.

Stress Relief Strategies:

1. Meditation:
   - Practice mindfulness meditation to calm the mind and reduce stress.

2. Deep Breathing:
  - Incorporate deep breathing exercises to promote relaxation and alleviate tension.

3. Progressive Muscle Relaxation (PMR):
  - Perform PMR to systematically relax different muscle groups and release physical tension.

4. Leisure Activities:
  - Engage in enjoyable leisure activities like reading, listening to music, or spending time in nature.

5. Social Support:
  - Maintain strong social connections for emotional support and companionship.

6. Adequate Sleep:
  - Prioritize sufficient and quality sleep to support overall well-being and reduce stress.

7. Time Management:
  - Effectively manage time to reduce feelings of overwhelm and stress.

Incorporating a balanced exercise routine and prioritizing stress relief are integral components of managing Graves' disease.

Natural herbs

Before diving into the details, it's crucial to know that herbal remedies should complement, not replace, conventional medical treatments. Always consult with healthcare professionals before integrating herbs into your wellness routine.

1. Lemon Balm (Melissa officinalis):

How to Use:
- Tea Infusion: Steep 1-2 teaspoons of dried lemon balm leaves in hot water for 5-10 minutes.
- Tincture: Consume 1-2 ml of lemon balm tincture up to three times daily.

Why it Works:
- Thyroid Regulation: Lemon balm may help modulate an overactive thyroid by influencing thyroid-stimulating hormone (TSH) levels.

- Calming Effect: Its gentle sedative properties can aid in stress reduction, potentially supporting Graves' disease management.

Precautions:
- Interactions: Consult with healthcare providers, especially if taking medications or experiencing drowsiness.
- Allergies: Exercise caution if allergic to plants in the Lamiaceae family (mint family).

2. Bugleweed (Lycopus virginicus):

How to Use:
- Infusion: Steep 1-2 teaspoons of dried bugleweed in hot water for 10-15 minutes.
- Tincture: Consume 2-4 ml of bugleweed tincture up to three times daily.

Why it Works:
- Thyroid Inhibition: Bugleweed may help inhibit the production of thyroid hormones, offering potential relief for hyperthyroid symptoms.
- Anti-inflammatory: Its anti-inflammatory properties can support overall thyroid health.

Precautions:

- Consultation: Discuss usage with healthcare providers, especially for those with hypothyroidism.
- Pregnancy: Avoid during pregnancy due to potential effects on thyroid function.

3. Motherwort (Leonurus cardiaca):

How to Use:
- Infusion: Steep 1-2 teaspoons of dried motherwort in hot water for 10-15 minutes.
- Tincture: Consume 2-4 ml of motherwort tincture up to three times daily.

Why it Works:
- Heart Support: Motherwort offers cardiovascular benefits, particularly relevant for those with Graves' disease.
- Nervine Tonic: Its calming effects can aid in managing stress and anxiety.

Precautions:
- Blood Pressure: Monitor blood pressure, as motherwort may affect it.
- Surgery: Discontinue use at least two weeks before scheduled surgery due to potential impact on blood pressure.

4. Ashwagandha (Withania somnifera):

How to Use:
- Powder: Mix 1/2 to 1 teaspoon of ashwagandha powder into warm milk or water.
- Capsules: Follow the recommended dosage on the supplement label.

Why it Works:
- Adaptogenic Qualities: Ashwagandha is an adaptogen, helping the body adapt to stress.
- Anti-inflammatory: Its anti-inflammatory properties may offer support for autoimmune conditions.

Precautions:
- Sensitivity: Start with a low dose to gauge individual sensitivity.
- Thyroid Function: Regularly monitor thyroid function due to potential interactions.

5. Hawthorn (Crataegus spp.):

How to Use:
- Tea Infusion: Steep 1-2 teaspoons of dried hawthorn berries in hot water for 10-15 minutes.
- Tincture: Consume 2-4 ml of hawthorn tincture up to three times daily.

Why it Works:
- Cardiac Support: Hawthorn supports cardiovascular health, crucial for those with Graves' disease.
- Anti-anxiety: Its calming properties contribute to stress reduction.

Precautions:
- Blood Pressure: Monitor blood pressure, as hawthorn may influence it.
- Medications: Consult healthcare providers, especially if taking medications.

6. Skullcap (Scutellaria lateriflora):

How to Use:
- Tea Infusion:bSteep 1-2 teaspoons of dried skullcap in hot water for 10-15 minutes.
- Tincture: Consume 2-4 ml of skullcap tincture up to three times daily.

Why it Works:
- Nervine Tonic: Skullcap offers nervine support, aiding in anxiety and stress management.
- Anti-inflammatory: Its anti-inflammatory properties contribute to overall well-being.

Precautions:
- Sedation: Skullcap may have mild sedative effects, so avoid combining with sedative medications.
- Pregnancy: Limited research during pregnancy, so consult with healthcare providers.

Incorporating these herbs into your routine requires mindfulness, individual observation, and collaboration with healthcare providers. Regular monitoring of thyroid function, stress levels, and overall well-being is crucial. While herbs can be valuable allies, they are part of a comprehensive approach that includes proper medical care, a balanced diet, and lifestyle adjustments.

Remember, everyone responds differently to herbs, so it's essential to listen to your body and seek professional guidance.

Managing Symptoms

Certainly, let's explore common symptoms associated with Graves' disease and simple strategies for managing each:

1. Hyperthyroidism Symptoms:

a. Rapid Heartbeat and Palpitations:
Management:
- Beta-blockers: Medications like propranolol can help regulate heart rate.
- Stress Management: Practice relaxation techniques to reduce anxiety.

b. Weight Loss and Increased Appetite:
Management:
- Nutrient-Dense Diet: Consume small, frequent meals with a focus on nutrient-rich foods.
- Consult a Dietitian: Seek guidance for maintaining a healthy weight.

c. Heat Sensitivity and Sweating:
Management:
- Cooling Strategies: Use fans, wear lightweight clothing, and stay hydrated.
- Avoid Excessive Heat: Limit exposure to hot environments.

2. Eye Symptoms (Graves' Ophthalmopathy):

a. Bulging Eyes (Exophthalmos):

Management:
- Eye Moisturizers: Use lubricating eye drops to relieve dryness.
- Sleep with Head Elevated: Reduce fluid accumulation around the eyes by sleeping with the head slightly elevated.

b. Double Vision:
Management:
- Eye Patches: Use an eye patch if double vision occurs, especially when reading or watching TV.
- Eye Exercises: Follow prescribed eye exercises to improve coordination.

c. Light Sensitivity:
Management:
- Sunglasses:bWear sunglasses to reduce sensitivity to bright lights.
- Artificial Tears: Use artificial tears to soothe irritated eyes.

3. Thyroid Eye Disease (TED) Symptoms:

a. Swelling and Redness:
Management:
- Cold Compresses: Apply cold compresses to reduce swelling.

- Topical Steroids: In severe cases, a doctor may prescribe steroids.

b. Pain and Discomfort:
Management:
- Pain Relievers: Over-the-counter pain relievers like acetaminophen can help alleviate discomfort.
- Avoid Smoking: Smoking can worsen eye symptoms; quitting is beneficial.

c. Blurred or Double Vision:
Management:
- Eye Exercises: Practice eye exercises recommended by an eye care professional.
- Vision Correction: Use corrective lenses as needed.

4. Emotional Symptoms:

a. Anxiety and Irritability:
Management:
- Mindfulness Practices: Engage in mindfulness meditation or deep breathing exercises.
- Regular Exercise: Physical activity can help manage stress.

b. Emotional Swings:

Management:
- Support Networks: Build a support system with friends, family, or a therapist.
- Express Yourself:bShare feelings with loved ones or in a journal.

5. Fatigue and Weakness:

a. Energy Conservation:
Management:
- Prioritize Rest: Ensure sufficient rest and prioritize sleep
- Delegate Tasks:* Delegate responsibilities to manage energy levels.

b. Balanced Diet:
Management:
- Nutrient-Rich Foods: Consume a well-balanced diet with a focus on vitamins and minerals.
- Hydration: Stay adequately hydrated for overall energy.

6. Skin and Hair Changes:

a. Dry Skin:
Management:

- Moisturize: Use hypoallergenic moisturizers to combat dryness.
- Avoid Hot Showers: Hot water can worsen dry skin; opt for lukewarm showers.

b. Hair Loss:
Management:
- Gentle Hair Care: Use a mild shampoo and avoid excessive heat styling.
- Supplements: Consult with a healthcare provider about supplements like biotin.

Managing Graves' disease involves a multi-faceted approach, including medical interventions, lifestyle adjustments, and self-care practices. Remember, these simple approaches are complementary and not a substitute for professional medical advice.

Chapter 7

Holistic Approaches to Hashimotos

Gluten-free and anti-inflammatory diets

In this chapter, we'll delve into the significance of adopting gluten-free and anti-inflammatory diets to foster well-being in the presence of Hashimoto's thyroiditis. These dietary choices aim to minimize inflammation and support your thyroid health.

Gluten-Free Diet: A Gentle Embrace for the Thyroid

Why Gluten-Free?
- Immune System Calming: For some individuals with Hashimoto's, gluten can trigger an immune response, exacerbating inflammation. Eliminating gluten may help calm the immune system.

Gluten-Free Choices:
- Whole Grains: Opt for gluten-free grains like rice, quinoa, and millet.
- Vegetables and Fruits: Embrace a colorful array of fruits and vegetables.
- Lean Proteins: Choose lean proteins such as poultry, fish, and legumes.
- Nuts and Seeds: Incorporate gluten-free nuts and seeds for added nutrients.

Recipes for a gluten free diet

1. Gluten-Free Spaghetti with Pesto and Grilled Chicken:

Ingredients:
- Gluten-free spaghetti
- 2 boneless, skinless chicken breasts
- 1 cup cherry tomatoes, halved
- 1/2 cup fresh basil leaves
- 1/4 cup pine nuts
- 1/2 cup grated Parmesan cheese
- 2 cloves garlic, minced
- 1/2 cup extra-virgin olive oil
- Salt and pepper to taste

Instructions:

1. Cook gluten-free spaghetti according to package instructions.
2. Season chicken breasts with salt and pepper, then grill until fully cooked.
3. In a food processor, combine basil, pine nuts, Parmesan cheese, garlic, and pulse.
4. While pulsing, gradually add olive oil until the pesto reaches a smooth consistency.
5. Toss cooked spaghetti with cherry tomatoes and pesto.
6. Slice grilled chicken and place on top.
7. Garnish with additional Parmesan and fresh basil.

2. Gluten-Free Tacos with Avocado Lime Crema:

Ingredients:
- Corn tortillas (gluten-free)
- 1 pound ground turkey or beef
- 1 tablespoon taco seasoning (gluten-free)
- 1 cup shredded lettuce
- 1 cup diced tomatoes
- 1 cup shredded cheddar cheese
- Avocado Lime Crema:
  - 1 ripe avocado
  - 1/4 cup Greek yogurt (gluten-free)
  - Juice of 1 lime
  - Salt and pepper to taste

Instructions:
1. In a skillet, brown the ground turkey or beef. Add taco seasoning and cook until fully done.
2. In a blender, combine avocado, Greek yogurt, lime juice, salt, and pepper. Blend until smooth.
3. Warm corn tortillas in a dry pan or microwave.
4. Assemble tacos with seasoned meat, lettuce, tomatoes, shredded cheese, and a dollop of avocado lime crema.

Anti-Inflammatory Diet: Soothing the Flames Within

Why Anti-Inflammatory?
- Reducing Systemic Inflammation: Chronic inflammation can worsen Hashimoto's symptoms. An anti-inflammatory diet focuses on foods that help lower inflammation throughout the body.

Anti-Inflammatory Choices:
- Fatty Fish: Include omega-3-rich fish like salmon and mackerel.
- Colorful Vegetables: Incorporate a variety of colorful vegetables for diverse antioxidants.

- Healthy Fats: Opt for olive oil, avocados, and nuts for anti-inflammatory fats.
- Turmeric and Ginger: These spices have natural anti-inflammatory properties.

Recipes for anti inflammatory diet

1. Anti-Inflammatory Turmeric Chickpea Curry:

Ingredients:
- 1 can chickpeas, drained and rinsed
- 1 tablespoon coconut oil
- 1 onion, diced
- 2 cloves garlic, minced
- 1 tablespoon fresh ginger, grated
- 1 tablespoon turmeric powder
- 1 teaspoon cumin
- 1 teaspoon coriander
- 1 teaspoon paprika
- 1 can diced tomatoes
- 1 can coconut milk (full-fat)
- Salt and pepper to taste
- Fresh cilantro for garnish

Instructions:
1. Heat coconut oil in a large pan over medium heat.

2. Add diced onion, minced garlic, and grated ginger. Sauté until fragrant.

3. Stir in turmeric, cumin, coriander, and paprika. Cook for 1-2 minutes.

4. Add chickpeas, diced tomatoes, and coconut milk. Simmer for 15-20 minutes.

5. Season with salt and pepper to taste.

6. Garnish with fresh cilantro before serving.

7. Serve over quinoa or brown rice.

2. Salmon and Kale Salad with Lemon-Turmeric Dressing:

Ingredients:
- 2 salmon fillets
- 4 cups kale, destemmed and chopped
- 1 cup cherry tomatoes, halved
- 1 avocado, sliced
- 1/4 cup pumpkin seeds (pepitas)
- Lemon-Turmeric Dressing:
  - Juice of 1 lemon
  - 2 tablespoons olive oil
  - 1 teaspoon turmeric powder
  - 1 teaspoon honey (optional)
  - Salt and pepper to taste

Instructions:

1. Season salmon fillets with salt and pepper. Grill or bake until cooked through.
2. In a large bowl, combine chopped kale, cherry tomatoes, avocado slices, and pumpkin seeds.
3. Whisk together lemon juice, olive oil, turmeric powder, honey (if using), salt, and pepper to create the dressing.
4. Flake the grilled salmon and add it to the salad.
5. Drizzle the lemon-turmeric dressing over the salad and toss gently.
6. Serve immediately.

Meal Planning Tips for Success:

1. Whole, Unprocessed Foods:
   - Prioritize whole, unprocessed foods to maximize nutrient intake and minimize potential inflammatory triggers.

2. Mindful Eating:
   - Practice mindful eating to savor flavors and support healthy digestion. Chew your food thoroughly.

3. Hydration:

- Stay well-hydrated with water, herbal teas, and infused water with slices of citrus or cucumber.

4. Listen to Your Body:
   - Pay attention to how your body responds to different foods. Adjust your diet based on your individual needs.

Exercise for Hashimotos

Acknowledging the hypothyroidism aspect of Hashimoto's, let's explore exercises that aim to stimulate metabolism and energy levels with a moderate to higher intensity. .

1. Dynamic Cardiovascular Activities:

a. Running or Jogging:
- Interval Running: Combine bursts of high-intensity running with slower recovery periods.
- Sprinting: Short sprints followed by moderate-paced jogging for an effective cardiovascular workout.

b. High-Intensity Interval Training (HIIT):

- Full-Body Workouts: Incorporate exercises like burpees, jumping jacks, and mountain climbers in intervals.

2. Strength Training for Metabolic Boost:

a. Compound Exercises:
- Deadlifts: Engages multiple muscle groups, promoting strength and metabolism.
- Squats and Lunges: Effective for lower body strength and overall metabolic stimulation.

b. High-Intensity Strength Workouts:
- Circuit Training: Combine strength exercises with minimal rest for an intense workout.

3. Individualized Approach:

a. Listen to Your Body:
- Fatigue Management: Adjust intensity and duration based on energy levels.
- Recovery Consideration: Ensure adequate rest and recovery between intense sessions.

b. Professional Guidance:
- Endocrinologist Input: Discuss exercise plans with your endocrinologist.

- Fitness Professional: Work with a trainer familiar with hypothyroid considerations.

Prioritizing sufficient sleep

Why Prioritize Sleep?
- Hormonal Regulation: Quality sleep supports the balance of hormones, including those related to thyroid function.
- Immune System Support: A well-rested body is better equipped to manage immune responses, crucial for autoimmune conditions.
- Energy Restoration: Hashimoto's patients often experience fatigue, making sufficient sleep essential for energy renewal.

Practical Tips for Quality Sleep:

Sleep Hygiene Practices:
- Consistent Schedule: Aim for a regular sleep-wake cycle, even on weekends.
- Optimal Sleep Environment: Create a cool, dark, and quiet bedroom conducive to rest.
- Digital Detox: Limit screen time before bedtime to reduce exposure to blue light.

Relaxation Techniques:
- Mindfulness Meditation: Calm the mind with mindfulness exercises before sleep.
- Progressive Muscle Relaxation (PMR):bRelease tension through systematic muscle relaxation.
- Aromatherapy: Use calming scents like lavender to promote relaxation.

Addressing Sleep Challenges with Hashimoto's:

Insomnia:
- Establish a Bedtime Routine: Create a calming routine before bed to signal to your body that it's time to wind down.
- **Cognitive Behavioral Therapy for Insomnia (CBT-I):** Consider therapeutic approaches to address insomnia patterns.

Fatigue Despite Sleep:
- Consult Healthcare Providers: Persistent fatigue may require adjustments in medication or further evaluation by healthcare professionals.
- Thyroid Hormone Optimization: Ensure thyroid medication is effectively supporting hormone levels.

Prioritizing sufficient sleep is a fundamental aspect of managing Hashimoto's thyroiditis. It's not just about the quantity but the quality of sleep that contributes to your overall well-being. As you weave the tapestry of your Hashimoto's journey, let restful sleep be a cornerstone, supporting your body's resilience and vitality. Sweet dreams await on the path to harmony.

Natural herbs

1. Ashwagandha (Withania somnifera):

How it Works:
- Adaptogenic Qualities: Ashwagandha is an adaptogen, helping the body adapt to stress and supporting overall well-being.
- Thyroid Function: Some studies suggest it may help balance thyroid hormones.

How to Use:
- Supplements:bAvailable in capsule or powder form. Follow recommended dosage on the product.

2. Holy Basil (Ocimum sanctum):

How it Works:
- Anti-Inflammatory: Holy Basil exhibits anti-inflammatory properties.

- Stress Reduction: Known for its stress-relieving benefits.

How to Use:
- Tea: Prepare a calming tea using dried holy basil leaves.
- Tinctures:bAvailable in liquid form; follow dosage recommendations.

3. **Turmeric (Curcuma longa):**

How it Works:
- Anti-Inflammatory:bCurcumin, the active compound in turmeric, has potent anti-inflammatory effects.
- Antioxidant: Acts as an antioxidant, supporting overall health.

How to Use:
- Golden Milk:bCombine turmeric with milk and other spices for a soothing beverage.
- Supplements:bCurcumin supplements are available; consult with a healthcare provider for proper dosage.

4. **Lemon Balm (Melissa officinalis):**

How it Works:
- Calming Effects: Lemon balm has calming and soothing properties.
- Thyroid Support: Some studies suggest potential benefits for thyroid health.

How to Use:
- Tea: Steep dried lemon balm leaves for a relaxing tea.
- Tinctures: Available in liquid form; follow dosage recommendations.

5. Bladderwrack (Fucus vesiculosus):

How it Works:
- Iodine Content: Contains iodine, essential for thyroid function.
- Anti-Inflammatory: Offers potential anti-inflammatory effects.

How to Use:
- Supplements: Available in capsules or powder form. Ensure proper iodine intake; consult with a healthcare professional.

Managing symptoms

1. Fatigue:

Management:
- Balanced Diet: Ensure a nutrient-rich diet with adequate vitamins and minerals.
- Regular Exercise: Incorporate moderate-intensity exercises to boost energy levels.
- Adequate Sleep: Prioritize sufficient and quality sleep for optimal rest and recovery.

2. Weight Gain:

Management:
- Balanced Diet: Focus on whole foods, lean proteins, and complex carbohydrates.
- Regular Exercise: Include both cardiovascular and strength training exercises.
- Thyroid Medication Adjustment: Consult with your healthcare provider for potential medication adjustments.

3. Sensitivity to Cold:

Management:

- Layer Clothing: Dress warmly, especially in colder temperatures.
- Warm Baths: Take warm baths to help maintain body temperature.
- Stay Active: Engage in regular physical activity to generate body heat.

4. Dry Skin:

Management:
- Hydration: Drink plenty of water to keep the skin hydrated.
- Moisturize: Use hypoallergenic moisturizers to prevent dryness.
- Avoid Hot Showers: Opt for lukewarm showers to prevent further skin dehydration.

5. Hair Loss

Management:

- Nutrient-Rich Diet:
  a. Include Biotin: Foods rich in biotin, such as eggs, nuts, and sweet potatoes, support hair health.
  b. Iron and Zinc: Ensure adequate intake through foods like lean meats, beans, and seeds.

- Supplements:
  a. Biotin Supplements:
  b. Iron and Zinc Supplements:I

- Gentle Hair Care:
a. Mild Shampoos: Use sulfate-free, gentle shampoos to avoid harsh chemicals.
  b. Avoid Heat Damage: Minimize the use of hot styling tools to prevent further stress on hair.

- Thyroid Medication Monitoring:
a. Regular Check-ups: Ensure thyroid medication is optimized and regularly monitored.
  b. Thyroid Hormone Levels: Maintain a balance with the help of your healthcare provider.

- Scalp Massage:
a. Stimulate Blood Flow: Regular, gentle scalp massages can promote blood circulation to the hair follicles.
b. Natural Oils: Consider using nourishing oils like coconut or argan during massages.

6. Changes in Menstrual Patterns:

1. Omega-3 Fatty Acids:

- Supplement: Consider omega-3 supplements like fish oil for their anti-inflammatory properties, potentially beneficial for hormonal balance.

2. Vitamin D:
- Supplement: Adequate vitamin D levels are crucial for hormonal health. Discuss with your healthcare provider to determine if supplementation is necessary.

3. Adaptogenic Herbs:
- Ashwagandha and Rhodiola: These adaptogenic herbs may support stress management and hormonal balance. Consult with your healthcare provider for appropriate dosages.

4. Magnesium:
- Supplement: Magnesium can help alleviate menstrual cramps and support overall hormonal function. Consult with your healthcare provider for suitable forms and dosages.

5. B Vitamins:
- B-complex Supplement: B vitamins, especially B6 and B12, play a role in hormonal regulation. Discuss with your healthcare provider for personalized supplementation.

6. Turmeric:
   - Incorporate into Diet: Turmeric's anti-inflammatory properties may contribute to overall well-being. Consider adding it to your diet or discussing supplementation with your healthcare provider.

7. Probiotics:
   - Promote Gut Health: Probiotics can positively impact gut health, potentially influencing hormonal balance. Choose a high-quality probiotic supplement or include probiotic-rich foods in your diet.

8. Agnus Castus (Chasteberry):
   - Herbal Supplement: Known for its potential to regulate menstrual cycles, Agnus Castus may be discussed with your healthcare provider for suitability.

9. Evening Primrose Oil:
   - Supplement: Some women find relief from menstrual symptoms with evening primrose oil, but individual responses vary. Consult with your healthcare provider before use.

Chapter 8

Holistic Approaches to Goiter

In this chapter, we will delve into holistic strategies for managing goiter, exploring a comprehensive approach that incorporates lifestyle adjustments, dietary considerations, and natural remedies. Goiter, often associated with thyroid imbalances, calls for a nuanced and holistic perspective to promote overall thyroid health. Let's explore practical and natural ways to address goiter and support thyroid well-being.

Dietary approaches, regular physical activity, and stress management.

Goiter, often linked to thyroid imbalances, benefits from a comprehensive approach. Embracing a balanced diet, regular physical activity, and effective stress management can contribute to overall thyroid health. Let's delve into each aspect:

Dietary Approaches:

- Iodine-Rich Foods: Incorporate iodine-rich foods like seaweed, dairy, and fish. However, consult with your healthcare provider to ensure proper iodine balance.

- Antioxidant-Rich Diet: Include fruits, vegetables, and whole grains to provide antioxidants that support thyroid health.

- Selenium Sources: Foods rich in selenium, such as Brazil nuts and sunflower seeds, may have benefits for thyroid function.

Regular Physical Activity:

- Aerobic Exercises: Engage in regular aerobic activities like walking, jogging, or cycling to promote overall cardiovascular health.

- Strength Training: Incorporate strength training exercises to support muscle health and metabolism.

- Yoga or Tai Chi: These activities can aid in stress reduction and may have positive effects on thyroid function.

Stress Management:

- Mindfulness Practices: Integrate mindfulness meditation or deep-breathing exercises into your routine to manage stress levels.

- Regular Breaks: Schedule short breaks throughout the day to alleviate stress and prevent burnout.
- Hobbies and Relaxation: Engage in activities you enjoy to promote relaxation and reduce the impact of chronic stress.

Hydration:
- Adequate Water Intake: Stay well-hydrated as water supports overall health, including thyroid function.

Limit Goitrogenic Foods:
- Moderation: Consume cruciferous vegetables like broccoli and cabbage in moderation, as they contain goitrogens that may affect thyroid function.

Importance of good hygiene

While good hygiene practices might not directly impact the development of goiter, maintaining hygiene is crucial for overall health and can indirectly contribute to managing goiter and supporting thyroid health. Here's how good hygiene plays a role:

111

1. Prevention of Infections:
   - Reducing Complications: Goiter, often associated with thyroid imbalances, may become more susceptible to infections. Good hygiene practices, such as regular handwashing, can help prevent infections that might complicate goiter conditions.

2. Supporting General Well-being:
   - Reducing Stress: Good hygiene contributes to overall well-being, and stress management is essential for thyroid health. Practices like regular bathing and skin care can be part of a stress-reducing routine.

3. Maintaining a Healthy Lifestyle:
   - Diet and Nutrition: Hygiene in food preparation and consumption is crucial for preventing illnesses that may exacerbate thyroid conditions. Following proper hygiene in dietary habits supports overall health.

4. Reducing Environmental Toxins:
   - Clean Living Spaces: A clean living environment reduces exposure to environmental toxins that may

affect thyroid function. Regular cleaning practices contribute to a healthier home environment.

5. Preventing Respiratory Infections:

- Thyroid and Immune System: A well-maintained respiratory hygiene routine helps prevent respiratory infections, indirectly supporting the immune system and thyroid health.

6. Medication Administration:

- Sterile Practices: If medication is part of goiter management, maintaining good hygiene during medication administration ensures sterile conditions, reducing the risk of complications.

7. Overall Health Promotion:

- Comprehensive Care: Managing goiter often requires a holistic approach. Incorporating good hygiene practices aligns with overall health promotion, contributing to a healthier lifestyle.

While good hygiene alone is not a direct treatment for goiter, it forms part of a holistic approach to maintaining health and preventing complications.

Natural herbs for managing goiter

1. Bugleweed (Lycopus virginicus):
- Thyroid Regulation: Bugleweed has been traditionally used to regulate thyroid function and reduce symptoms of hyperthyroidism, which can sometimes contribute to goiter.

2. Lemon Balm (Melissa officinalis):
- Calming Effects: Lemon balm may have calming effects and could be beneficial for those with goiter related to stress. It's often used to support the nervous system.

3. Guggul (Commiphora wightii):
- Anti-inflammatory: Guggul has anti-inflammatory properties and may be beneficial for managing inflammation associated with thyroid conditions.

4. Turmeric (Curcuma longa):
- Anti-inflammatory and Antioxidant: Turmeric's active compound, curcumin, has anti-inflammatory and antioxidant properties that may support overall thyroid health.

5. Coleus Forskohlii:

- Forskolin Content: Forskolin, found in Coleus forskohlii, has been studied for its potential to support thyroid function and promote a balance of thyroid hormones.

8. Holy Basil (Ocimum sanctum):

- Adaptogenic and Antioxidant: Holy basil is an adaptogen with antioxidant properties, potentially supporting the body's response to stress and overall thyroid health.

Managing Symptoms

1. Difficulty Swallowing

- Hydrate Adequately: Ensure you stay well-hydrated throughout the day.
- Modify Food Texture: Opt for softer or more liquid-based foods.
- Small, Frequent Meals: Choose smaller, more frequent meals to make swallowing easier.

2. Fatigue

- Prioritize Sleep: Ensure sufficient and quality sleep each night.

- Balanced Diet: Consume a well-balanced diet with a mix of nutrients.
- Light Exercise: Engage in light and regular physical activity to boost energy levels.

3. Visible Swelling or Lump

- Cool Compress: Apply a cool compress to reduce swelling and discomfort.
- Neck Exercises: Gentle neck exercises may help improve flexibility and reduce tension.
- Iodine-Rich Foods: If appropriate, include iodine-rich foods in your diet.

4. Coughing or Hoarseness

- Throat Lozenges: Use throat lozenges to soothe irritation.
- Hydration: Drink warm beverages to keep the throat moist.
- Voice Rest: Give your voice regular breaks, especially if experiencing hoarseness.

5. Difficulty Breathing

- Maintain Good Posture: Sit or stand upright to support optimal breathing.

- Breathing Exercises: Practice deep breathing exercises for respiratory support.

- Avoid Triggers: Identify and avoid environmental triggers that may worsen breathing difficulties.

6. Changes in Voice

- Voice Rest: Give your voice regular breaks to prevent strain.

- Stay Hydrated: Drink plenty of water to keep vocal cords lubricated.

- Throat Coat Tea: Consider herbal teas with soothing properties for the throat.

Chapter 9

Holistic Approaches to Thyroiditis Tranquility

In this chapter, we explore holistic strategies for managing thyroiditis, emphasizing tranquility as a cornerstone for well-being. Thyroiditis, inflammation of the thyroid gland, can significantly impact one's physical and emotional state. By adopting a holistic approach that encompasses lifestyle adjustments, mindful practices, and natural remedies, individuals can cultivate a sense of tranquility to complement traditional medical interventions. Let's delve into practical and calming methods to support those navigating thyroiditis, promoting a harmonious balance between the body and mind.

Anti-inflammatory dietary strategies

In managing thyroiditis, adopting an anti-inflammatory diet can be a valuable component of a holistic approach. Here are dietary strategies that may help reduce inflammation:

1. Omega-3 Fatty Acids:
   - Sources: Fatty fish (salmon, mackerel), flaxseeds, chia seeds, walnuts.
   - Why: Omega-3s have anti-inflammatory properties and support overall immune health.

2. Turmeric and Ginger:
   - Usage: Incorporate turmeric and ginger into meals or consume as teas.
   - Why: Curcumin in turmeric and gingerol in ginger possess potent anti-inflammatory effects.

3. Colorful Vegetables:
   - Include: A variety of colorful vegetables (broccoli, kale, bell peppers, carrots).
   - Why: Rich in antioxidants, vitamins, and minerals that combat inflammation.

4. Berries:
   - Include: Blueberries, strawberries, raspberries.
   - Why: Berries are rich in antioxidants that help reduce inflammation.

5. Probiotics:

- Sources: Yogurt, kefir, sauerkraut, kimchi.
- Why: Support gut health, which is linked to immune function and inflammation.

6. Healthy Fats:
- Include: Avocado, olive oil, nuts.
- Why: Monounsaturated fats have anti-inflammatory properties.

7. Whole Grains:
- Choose: Quinoa, brown rice, oats.
- Why: Provide fiber and nutrients without causing inflammation.

8. Green Tea:
- Usage: Drink green tea regularly.
- Why: Contains catechins, which have anti-inflammatory and antioxidant effects.

9. Avoid Processed Foods:
- Limit: Processed foods, refined sugars, and trans fats.
- Why: These can contribute to inflammation and negatively impact overall health.

10. Hydrate with Water:
- Tip: Drink plenty of water throughout the day.

- Why: Hydration supports overall health and aids in the elimination of toxins.

Natural herbs

1. Siberian Ginseng (Eleutherococcus senticosus):
- Usage: Often available in supplement form.
- Why: Adaptogenic herb that may help the body cope with stress.

2. Nettle (Urtica dioica):
- Usage: Can be consumed as a tea or in supplement form.
- Why: Rich in nutrients and may have anti-inflammatory effects.

3. Guggul (Commiphora wightii):
- Usage: Available as a supplement.
- Why: Anti-inflammatory properties may be beneficial for thyroid health.

4. Coleus Forskohlii:
- Usage: Typically taken as a supplement.

- Why: Contains forskolin, which may support thyroid function.

Conclusion

Recap of key holistic strategies for each thyroid condition.

Hypothyroidism:

1. Dietary Approach:
   - Focus on iodine-rich foods, selenium, and a balanced diet.
   - Consider incorporating sea vegetables like seaweed.

2. Lifestyle Adjustments:
   - Prioritize sleep for hormonal balance.
   - Engage in regular exercise to boost metabolism.

3. Supplements:
   - Consider supplements like vitamin D and omega-3 fatty acids.

Hyperthyroidism:

1. Anti-Inflammatory Diet:

- Emphasize foods rich in antioxidants and anti-inflammatory properties.

2. Stress Management:
   - Practice stress-reduction techniques, including mindfulness and yoga.

3. Herbal Support:
   - Explore herbs like lemon balm and bugleweed for thyroid balance.

Graves' Disease:

1. Anti-Inflammatory Diet:
   - Follow an anti-inflammatory diet with nutrient-dense foods.

2. Stress Reduction:
   - Prioritize stress management for immune system support.

3. Natural Remedies:
   - Consider herbs like ashwagandha and guggul for immune modulation.

Hashimoto's Thyroiditis:

1. Gluten-Free Diet:
   - Adopt a gluten-free diet to manage autoimmune responses.

2. Anti-Inflammatory Foods:
   - Emphasize foods with anti-inflammatory properties, including turmeric.

3. Lifestyle Modifications:
   - Manage stress through relaxation techniques and sufficient sleep.

Thyroiditis

1. Anti-Inflammatory Diet:
   - Include omega-3 fatty acids, turmeric, and colorful vegetables.

2. Herbal Support:
   - Explore herbs like ashwagandha, bugleweed, and lemon balm.

3. Lifestyle Harmony:
   - Prioritize stress reduction through mindful practices and regular exercise.

Dear Reader,

I sincerely hope this guide empowers you on your journey to thyroid health. Each holistic strategy is a step toward creating balance and well-being. Remember, individual responses may vary, so consult with healthcare professionals for personalized advice.

If you find this guide valuable, I kindly ask for your support. Your feedback is invaluable, and I would be grateful for a kind review and a good rating. Thank you for entrusting me with a part of your wellness journey.

Wishing you health and tranquility,

Printed in Great Britain
by Amazon